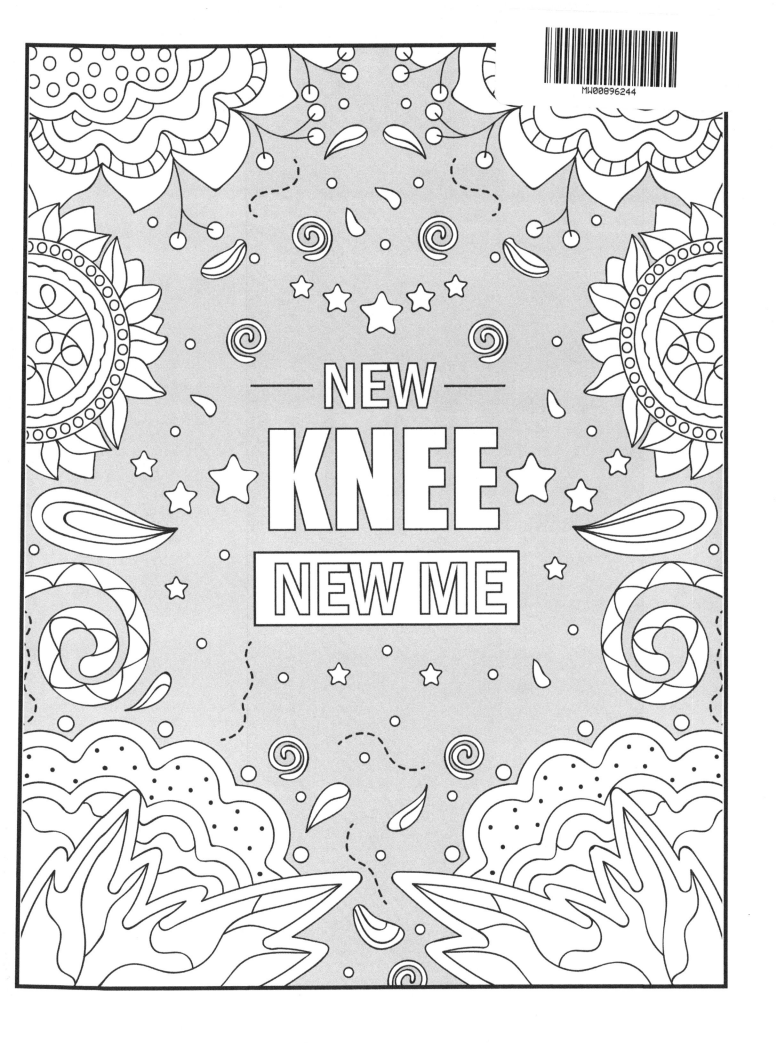

We would like to thank you personally for purchasing this book. This coloring book is a collection of 20+ funny and relatable Knee Surgery Coloring Pages.

At Sandesh Bogati Publishing we understand that having a Knee surgery can be tough. So, to let you add some fun and relaxation to your Knee surgery recovery we have created this coloring book.

Published by Sandesh Bogati Publishing

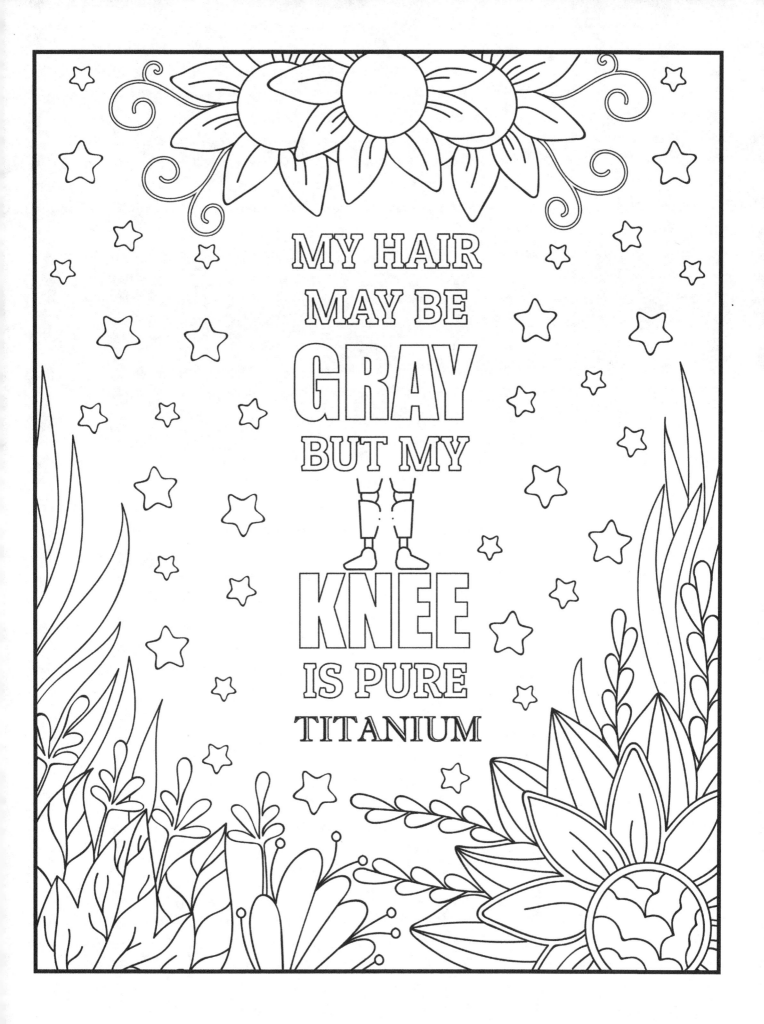

MY HAIR MAY BE GRAY BUT MY KNEE IS PURE TITANIUM

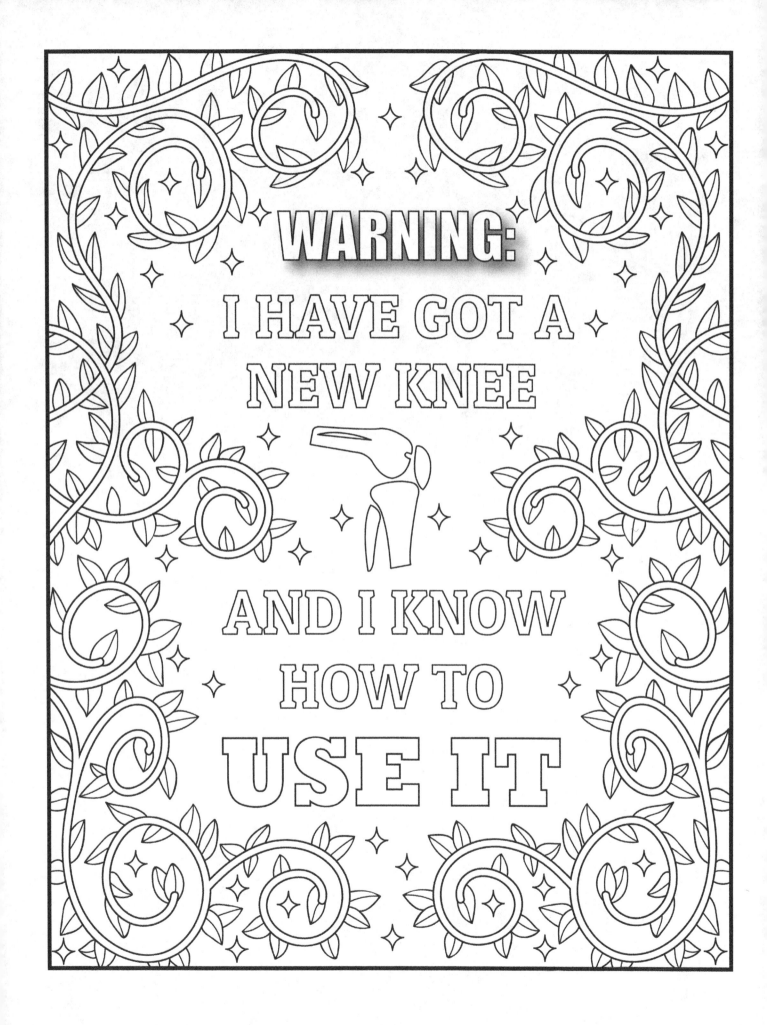

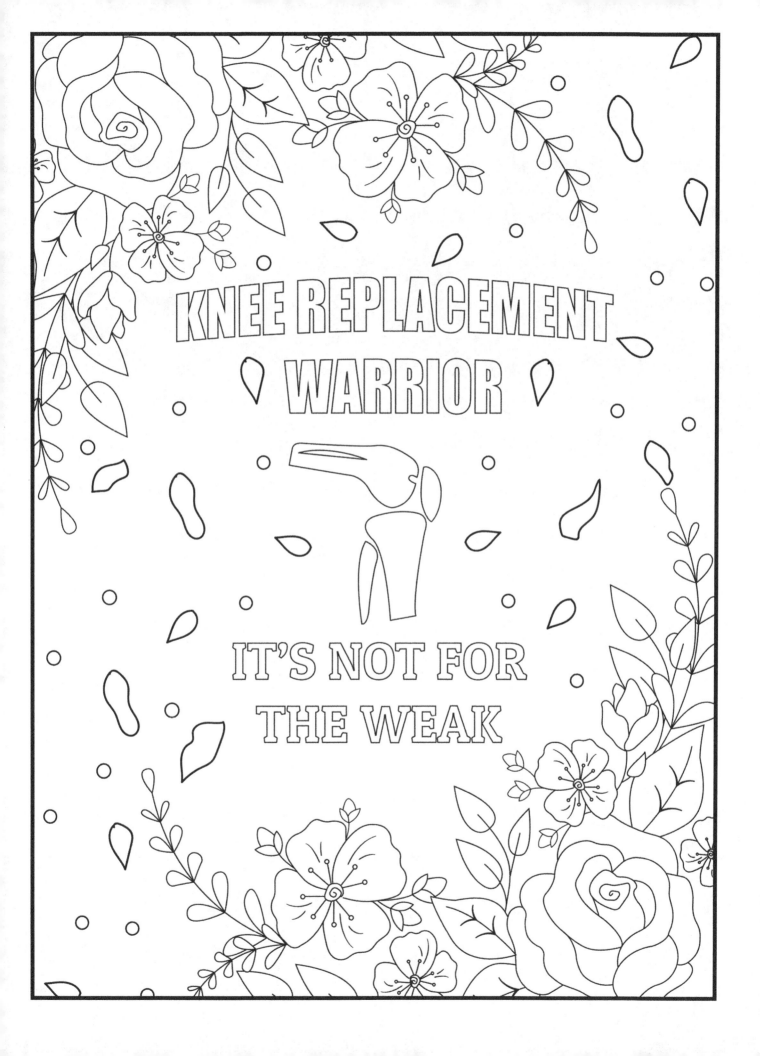

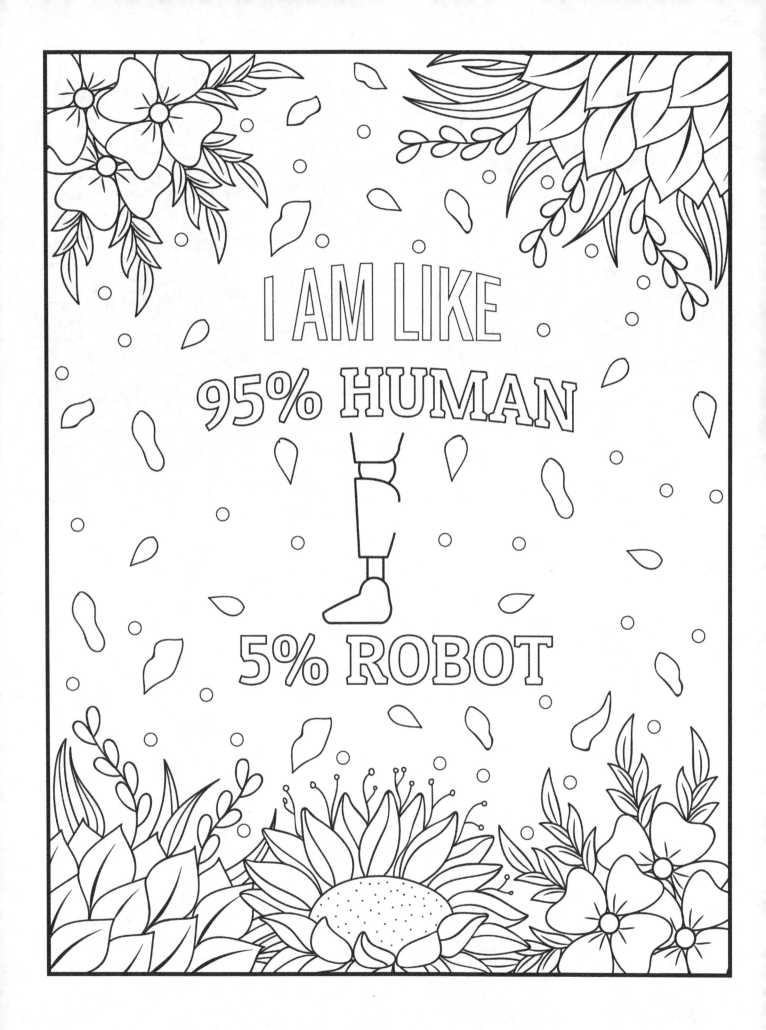

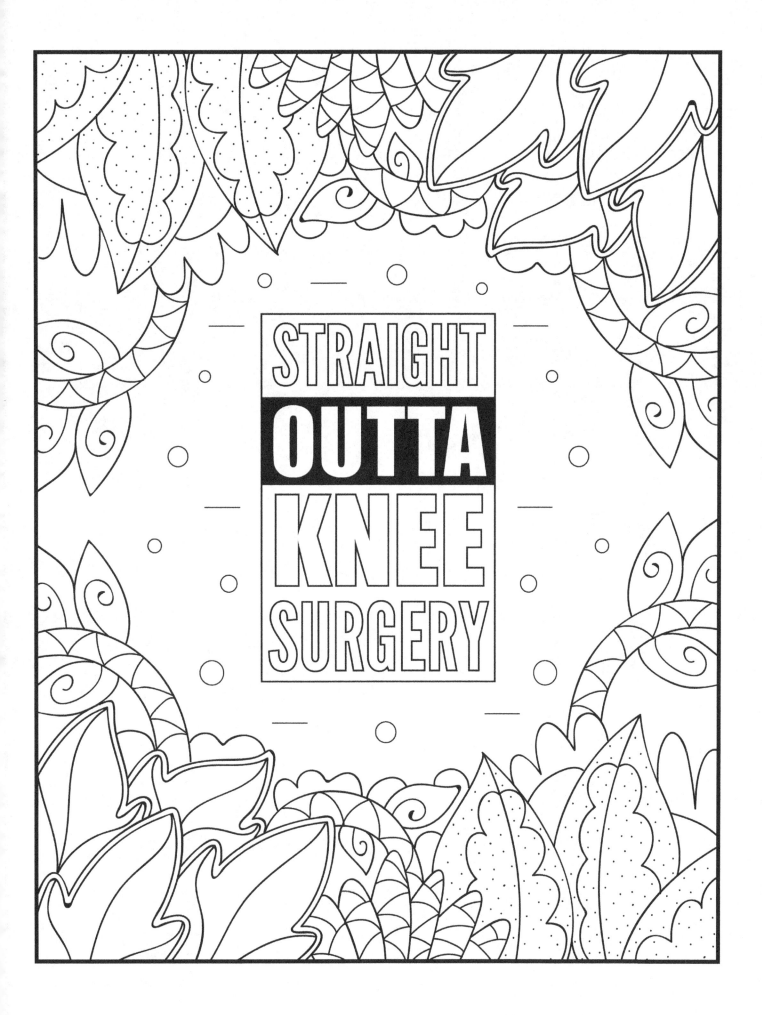

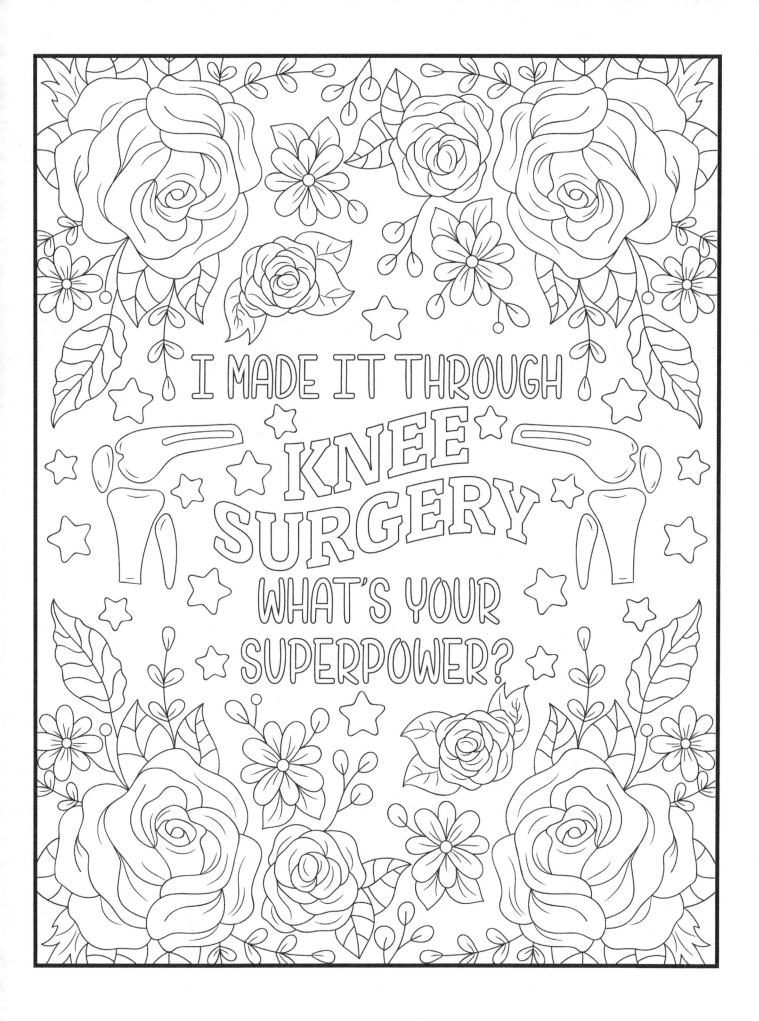

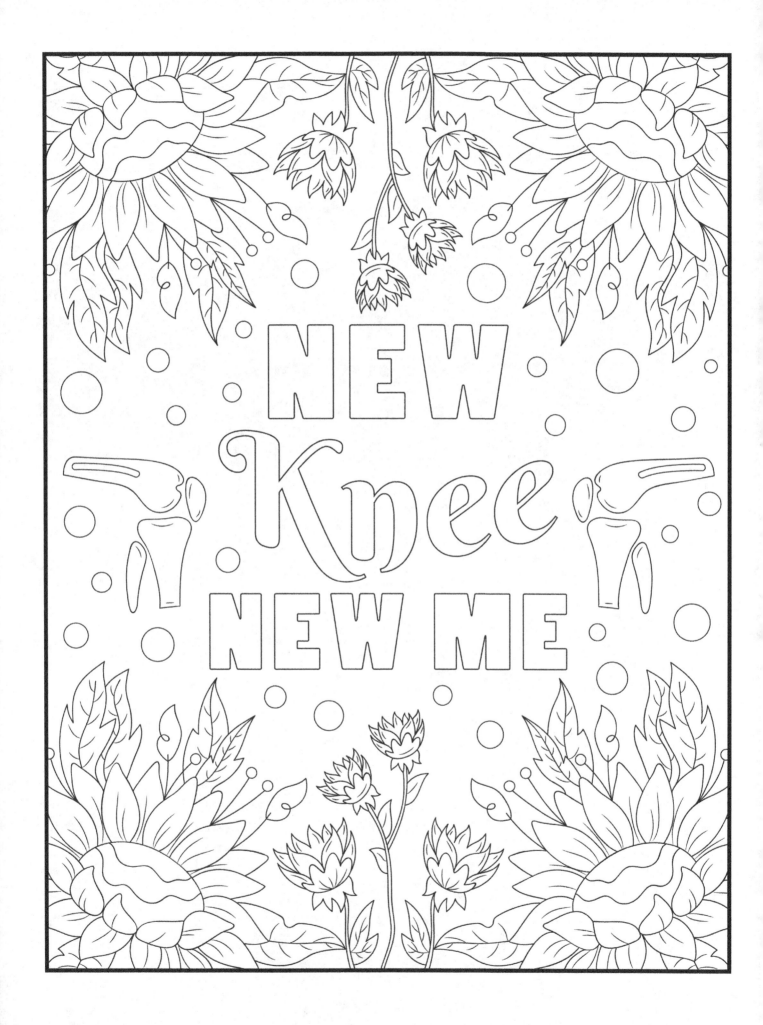

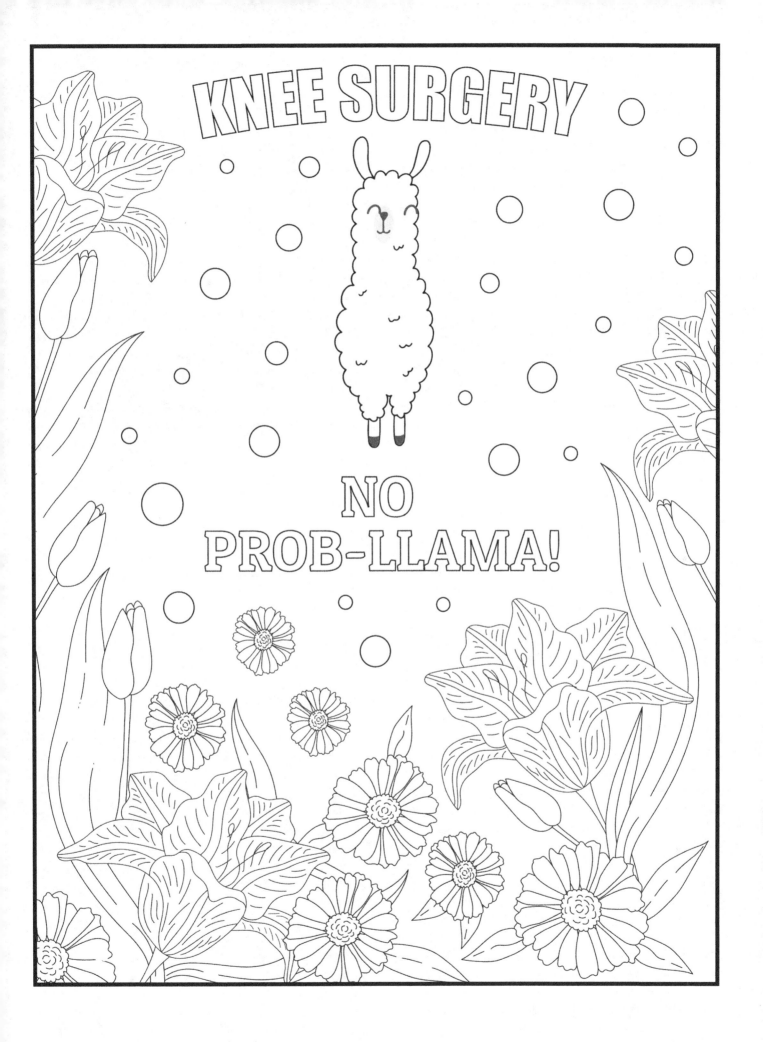

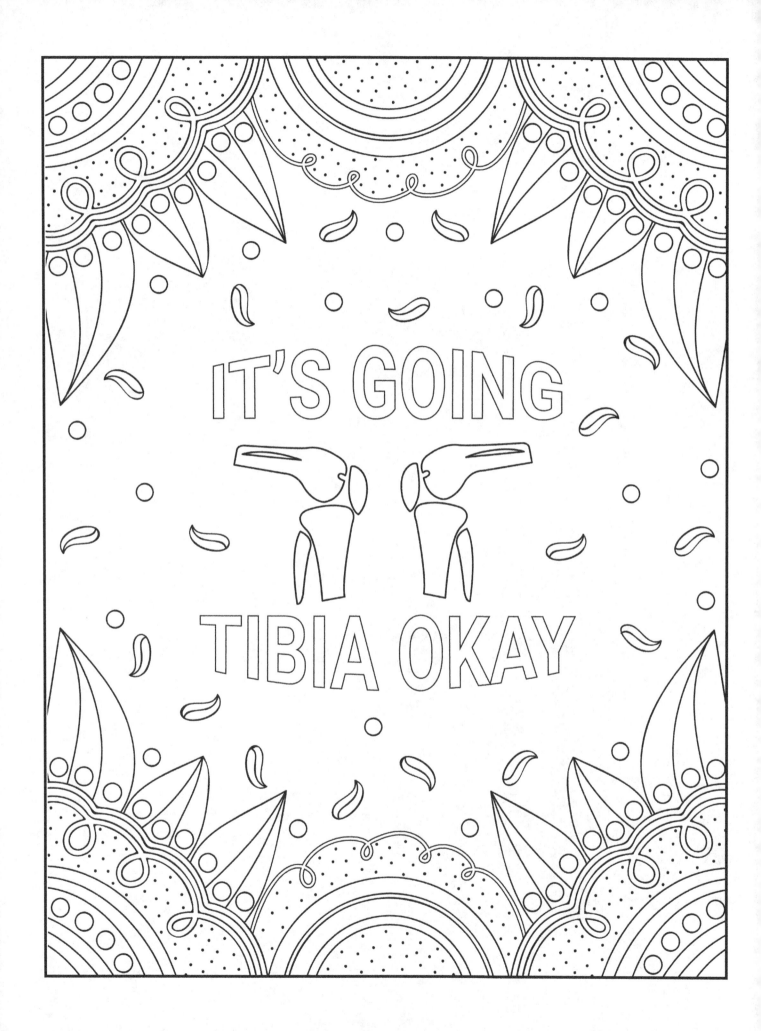

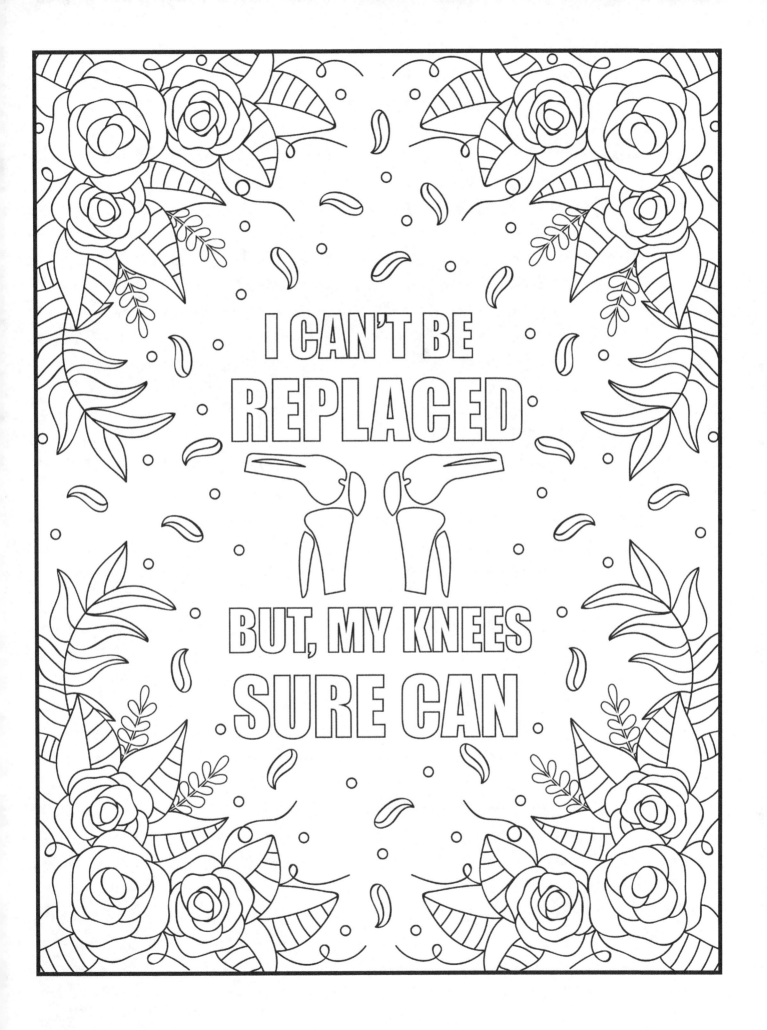

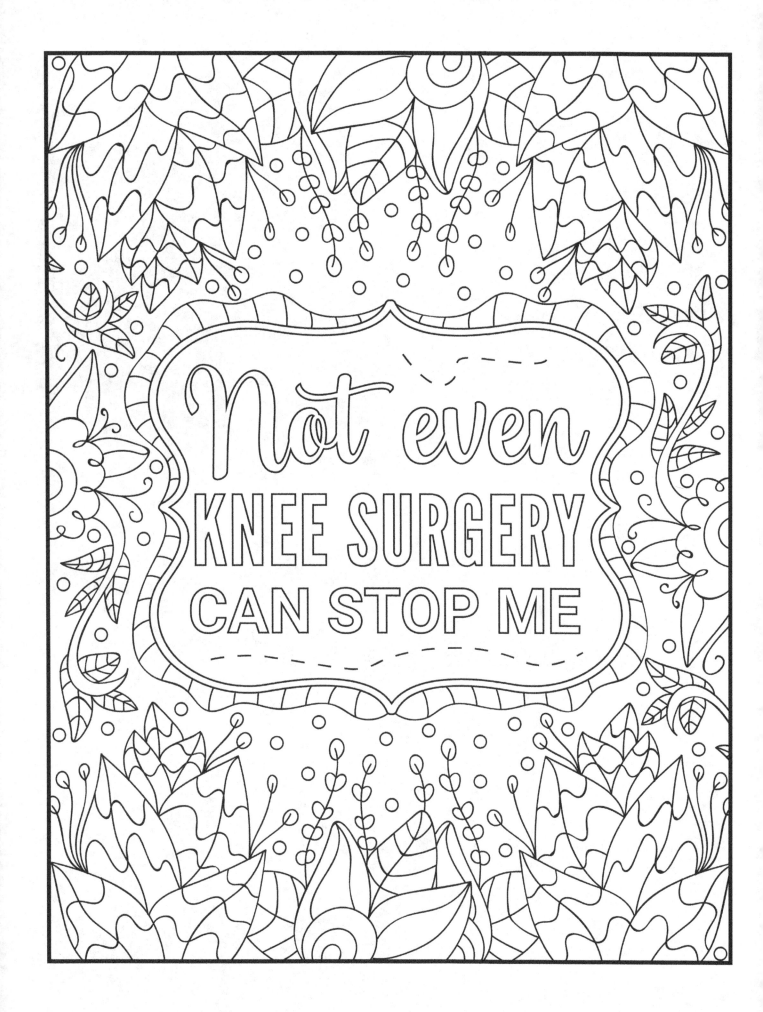

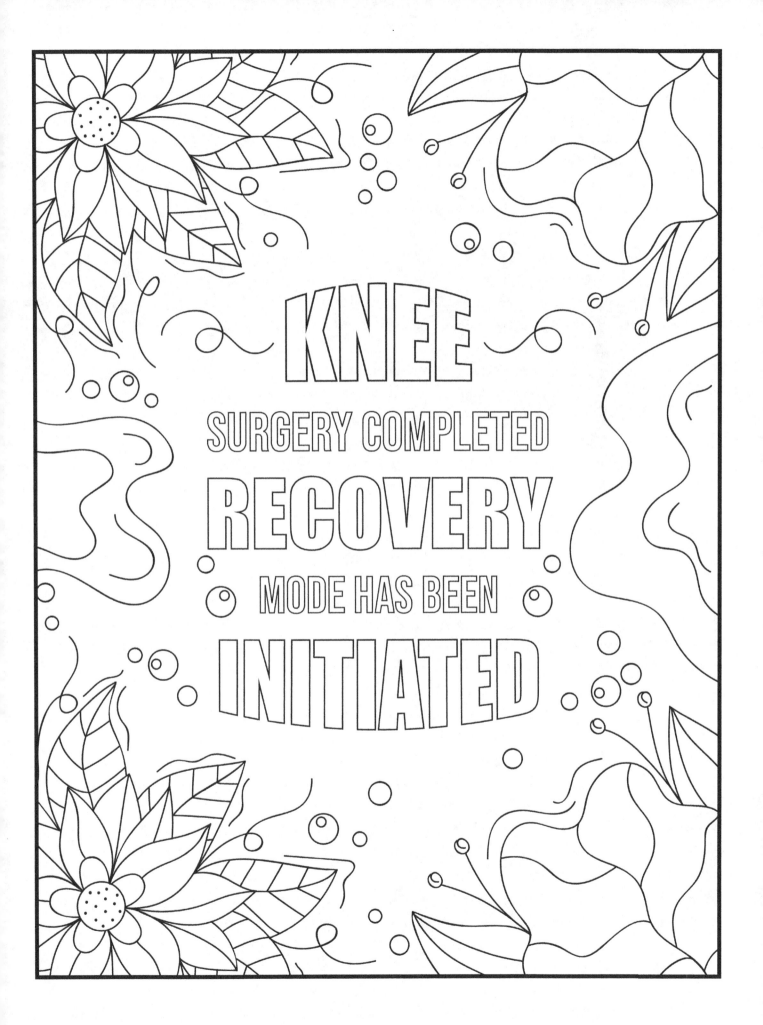

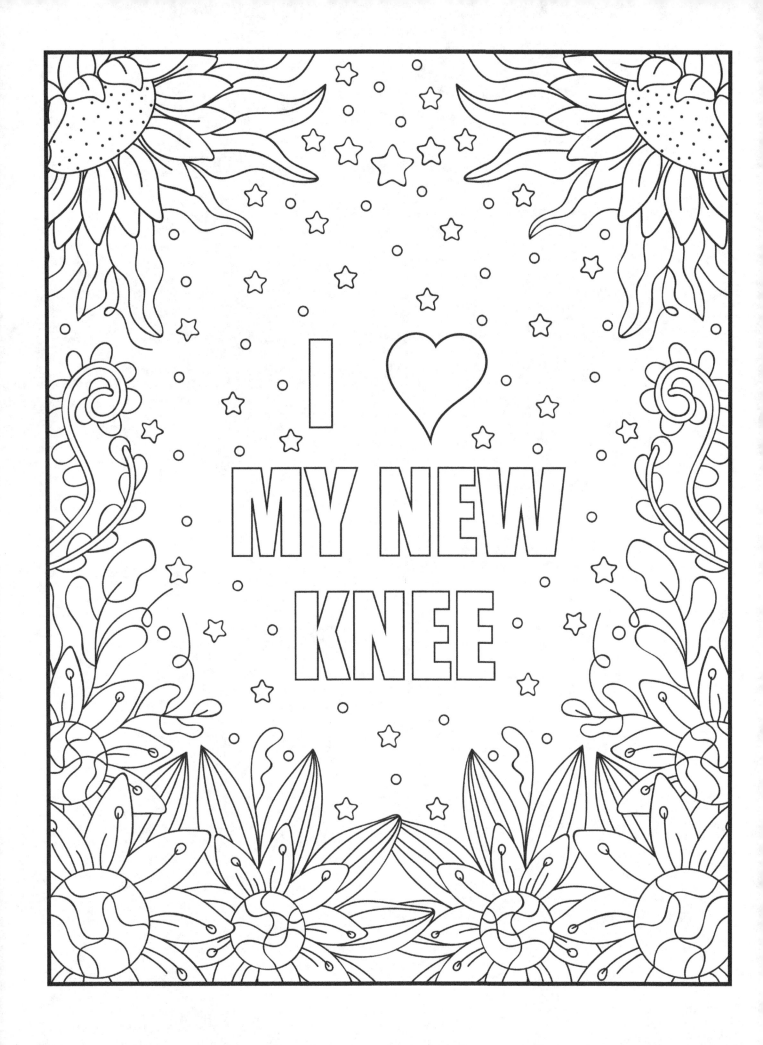

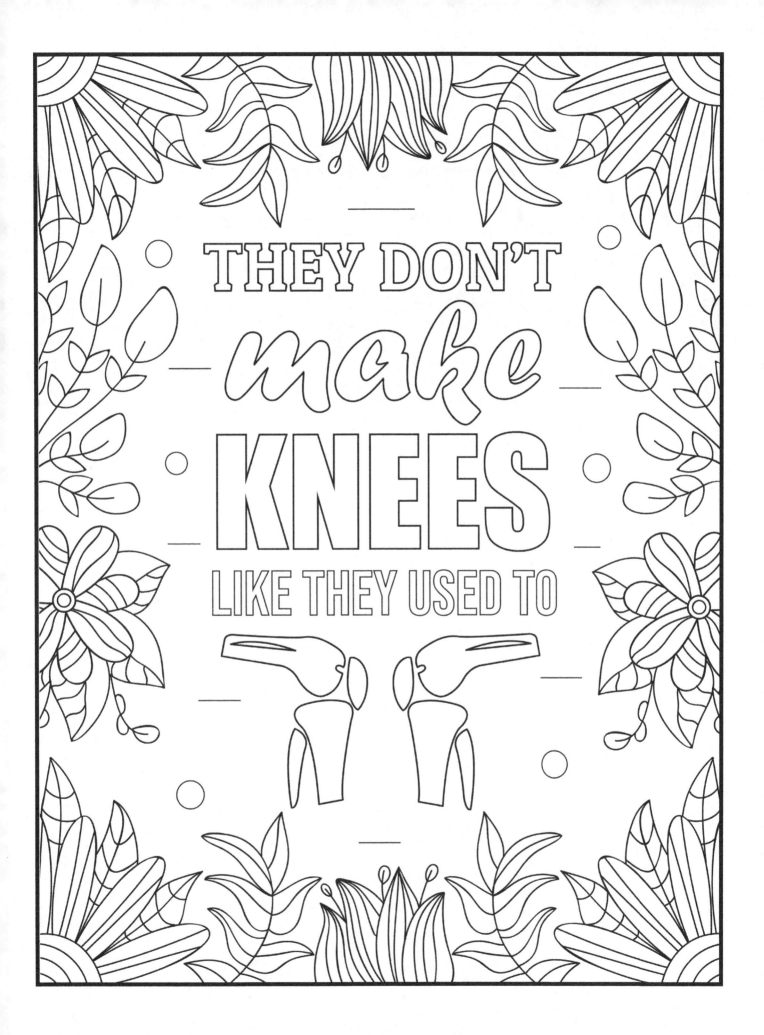

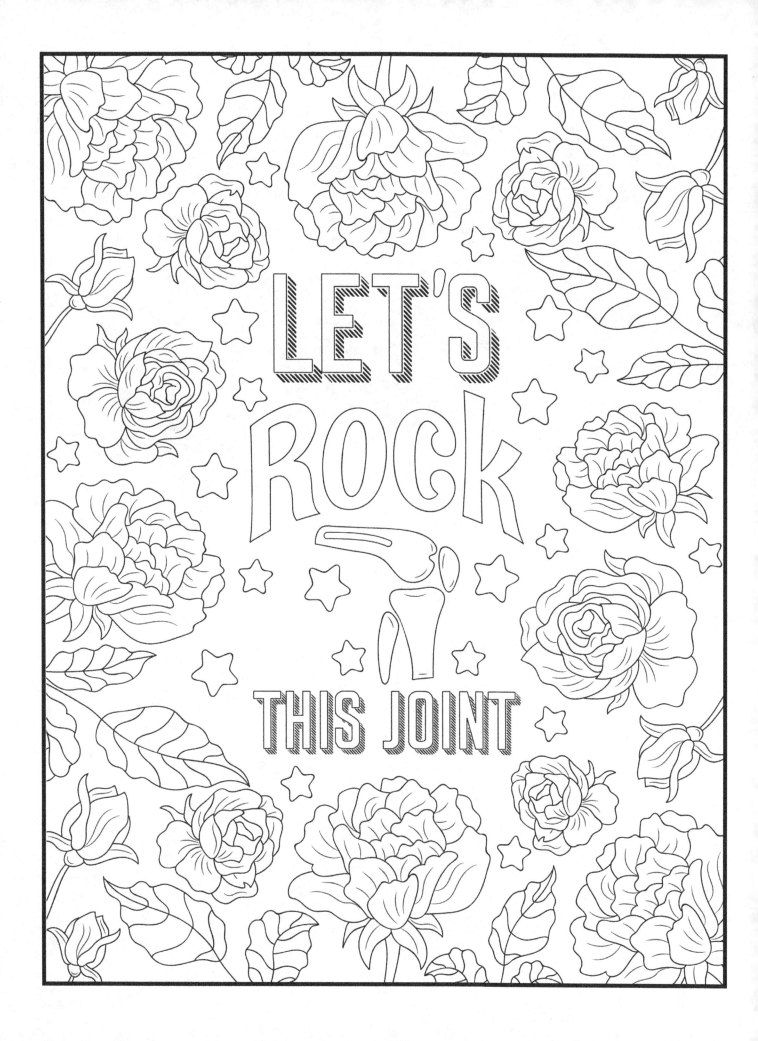

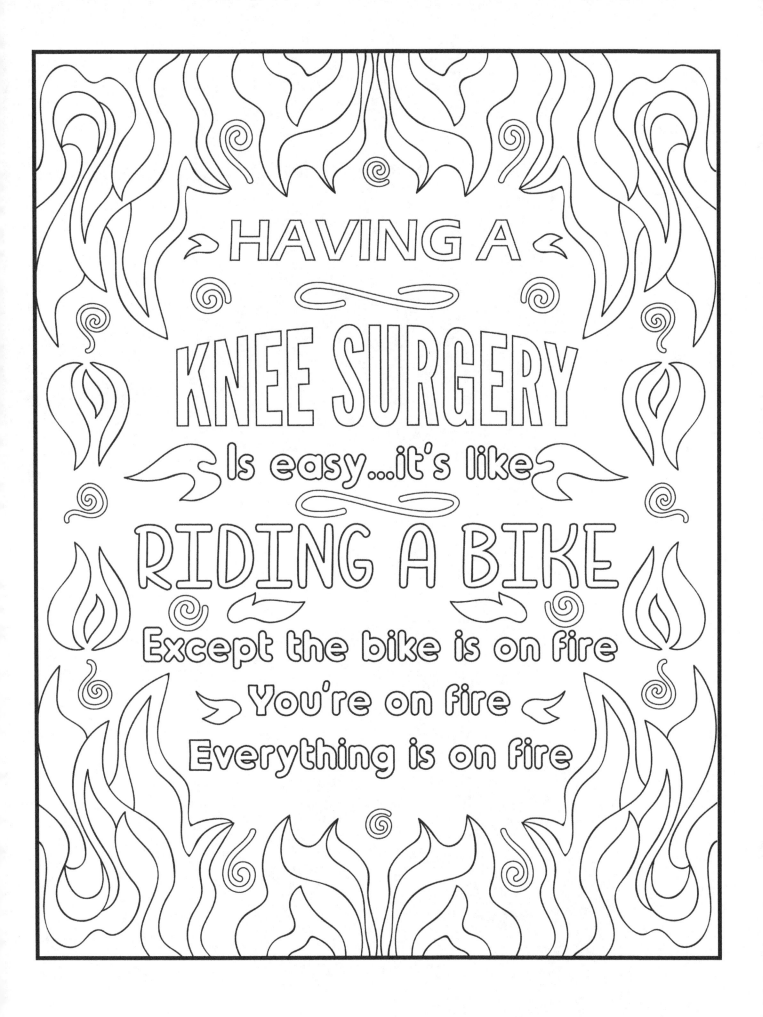

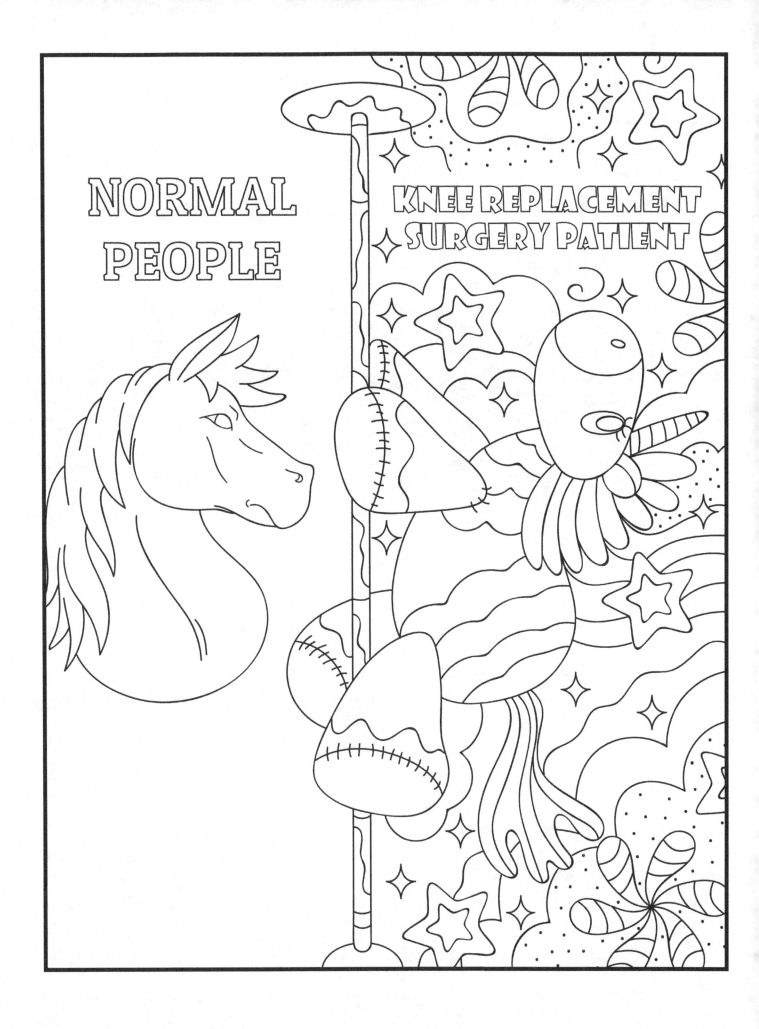

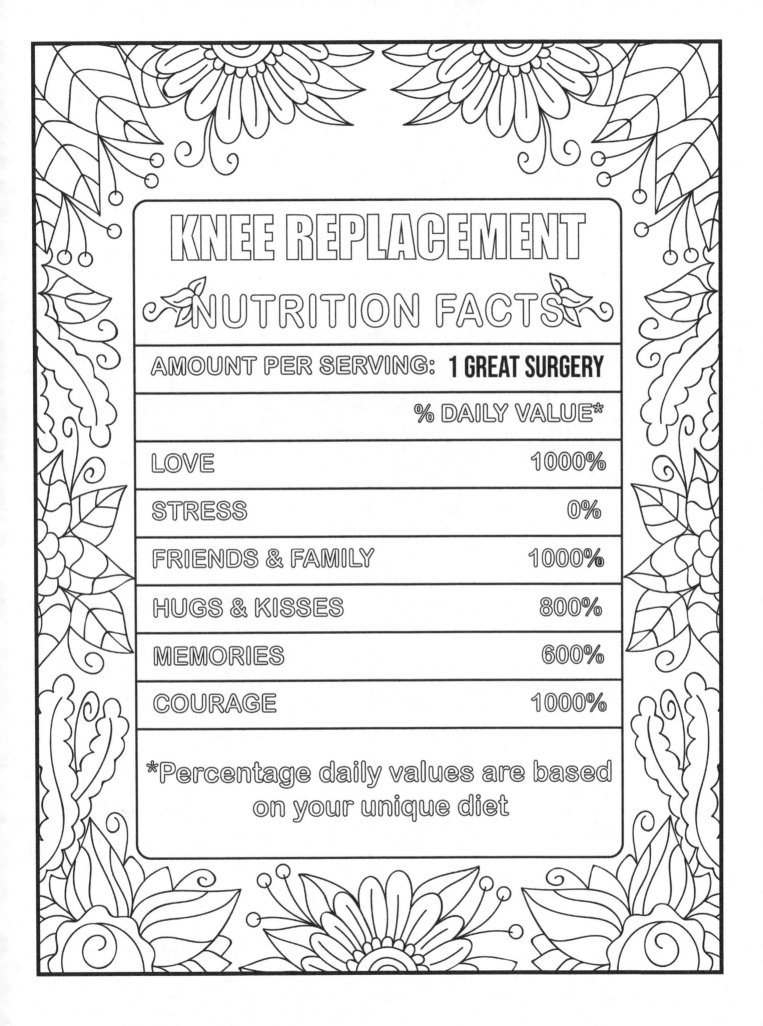

KNEE REPLACEMENT

NUTRITION FACTS

AMOUNT PER SERVING: 1 GREAT SURGERY

% DAILY VALUE*

LOVE	1000%
STRESS	0%
FRIENDS & FAMILY	1000%
HUGS & KISSES	800%
MEMORIES	600%
COURAGE	1000%

*Percentage daily values are based on your unique diet

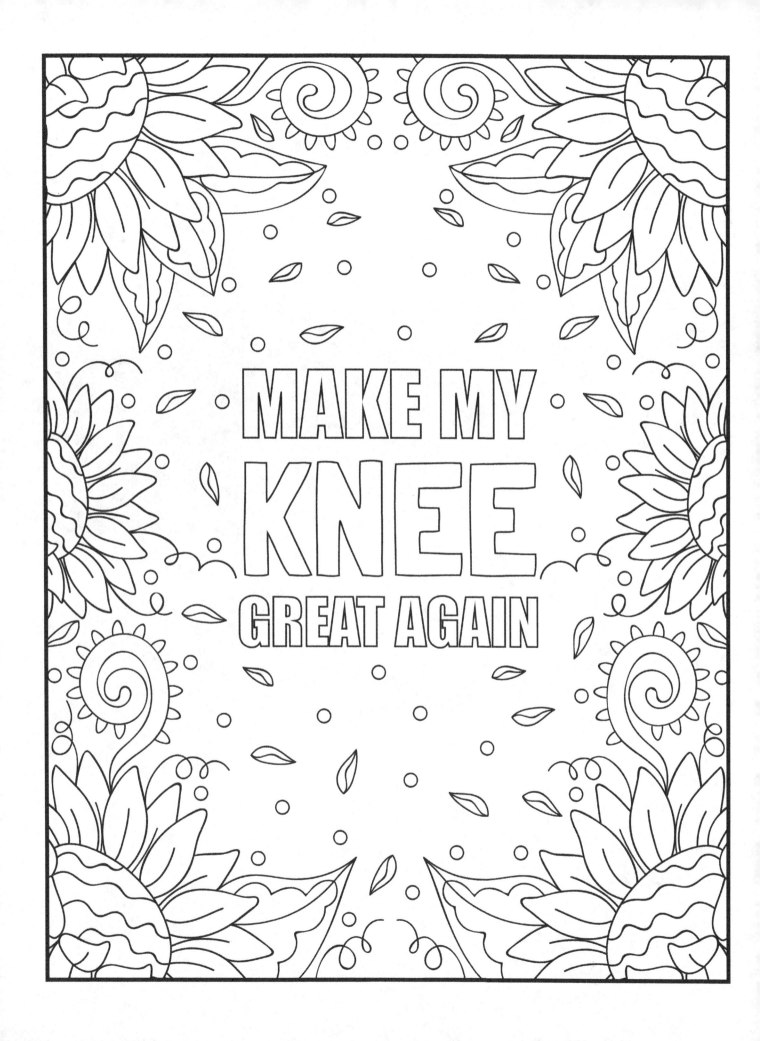

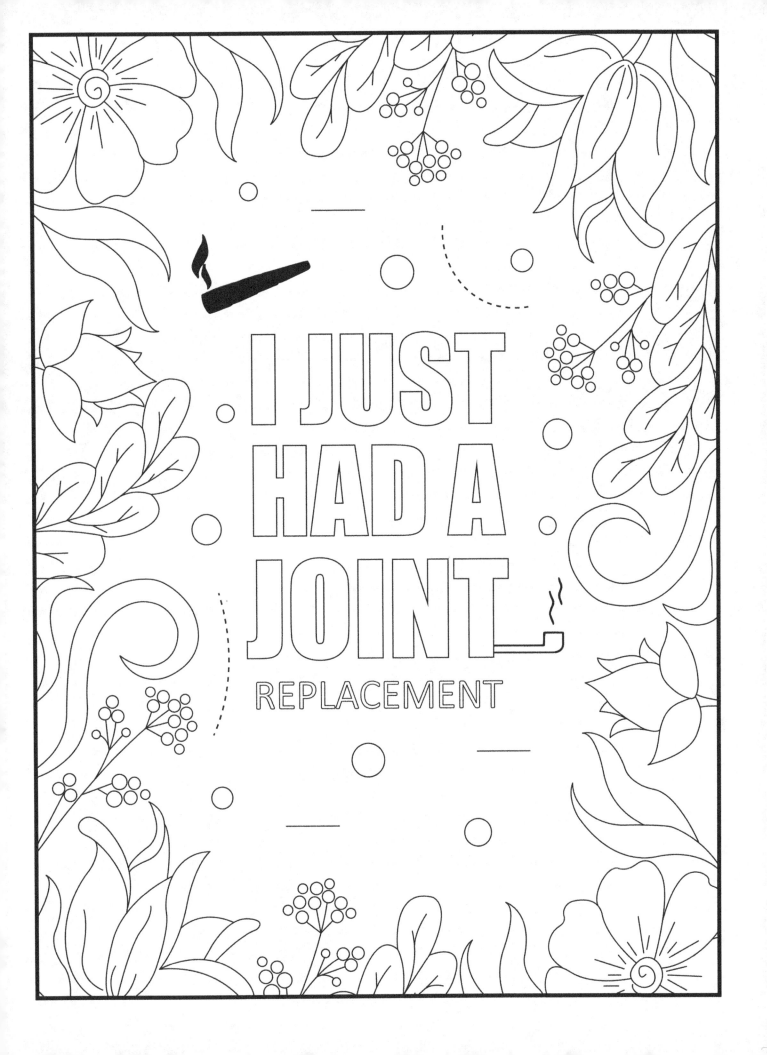

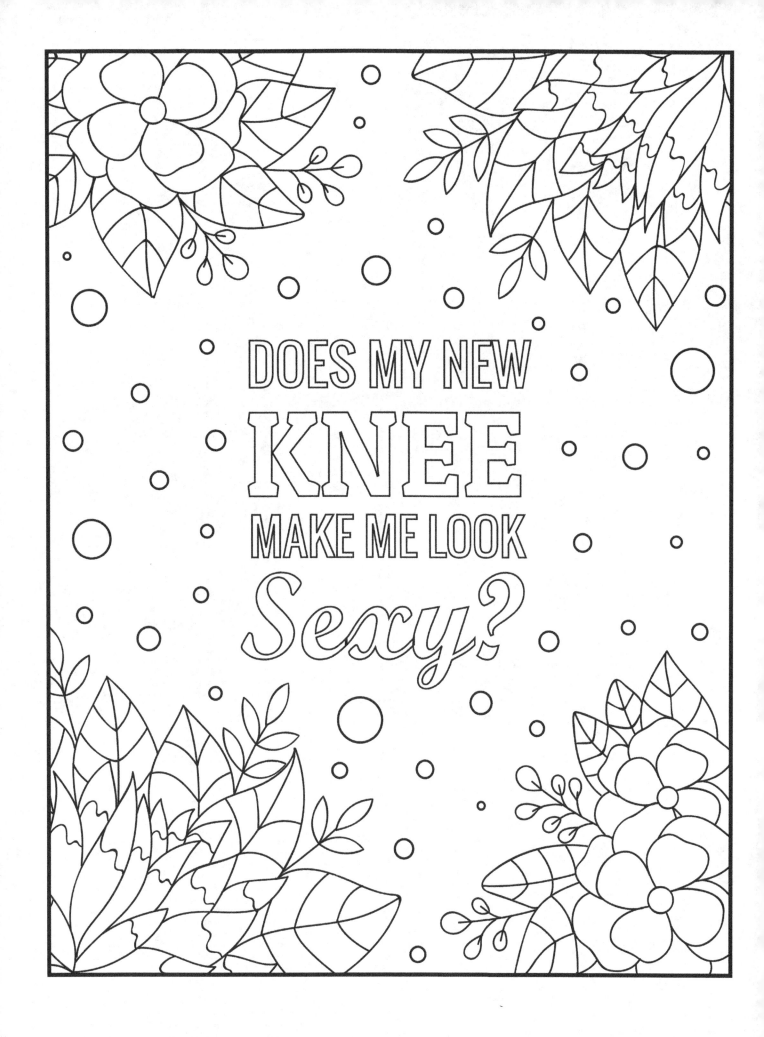

Made in the USA
Coppell, TX
31 October 2023

23647485R00031